Metabolic Flexibility Diet Guide for Beginners

Key Components of the Metabolic Flexibility Diet

By

Caelan Murray

Table of Contents

CHAPTER 1

Introduction

In the complex tapestry of human physiology, the concept of metabolic flexibility emerges as a pivotal factor influencing overall health and well-being. This introduction serves as the gateway to understanding the intricacies of metabolic flexibility and delves into its significance within the broader context of human metabolism.

1.1 Overview of Metabolic Flexibility

Metabolic flexibility, a term gaining increasing recognition in scientific and health circles, refers to the body's capacity to adapt and efficiently utilize different fuel sources for energy production. At its core, metabolic flexibility encompasses the dynamic ability of the body to switch between carbohydrates and fats as primary sources of energy, depending on the physiological demands and availability of nutrients.

1.2 Importance of Diet in Metabolic Flexibility

The interplay between diet and metabolic flexibility takes center stage in this exploration. Diet, as a modifiable factor, emerges as a potent influencer of metabolic adaptability. This impact of dietary choices on the body's ability to efficiently utilize and switch between energy substrates. It sheds light on the pivotal role played by macronutrients—carbohydrates, fats, and proteins—in sculpting the metabolic landscape.

CHAPTER 2

Understanding Metabolic Flexibility

Embarking on the journey to understand metabolic flexibility requires a nuanced exploration of the fundamentals of metabolism and the myriad factors that intricately weave together to shape the body's ability to adapt and optimize energy utilization.

2.1 Basics of Metabolism

Metabolism, often likened to the body's intricate engine, is a dynamic and finely regulated process responsible for the conversion of food into energy. From the catabolic breakdown of macronutrients into simpler molecules to the anabolic synthesis of complex cellular structures, the intricate dance of enzymes and molecular messengers orchestrates a symphony essential for life.

The journey through glycolysis, the citric acid cycle, and oxidative phosphorylation unveils the energy currency of the cell—adenosine triphosphate (ATP).

2.2 Factors Influencing Metabolic Flexibility

Metabolic flexibility, although rooted in the core machinery of metabolism, is a dynamic trait influenced by an array of factors.

The first facet explored is the genetic underpinning of metabolic flexibility. While individuals inherit a genetic blueprint that influences their metabolic tendencies, the interplay between genes and environmental factors emerges as a key determinant. Epigenetic modifications, influenced by lifestyle and environmental exposures, add an additional layer of complexity to the genetic landscape.

Diving deeper, the impact of age on metabolic flexibility comes into focus. As the body undergoes natural physiological changes over the lifespan, such as alterations in hormonal profiles and changes in body composition, the adaptability of metabolism can be influenced. Understanding how metabolic flexibility evolves across different life stages is crucial for tailoring dietary and lifestyle interventions.

Environmental factors, encompassing diet, physical activity, and stress, play a pivotal role in shaping metabolic flexibility. The nutritional composition of one's diet, the intensity and type of physical activity, and the stressors encountered in daily life collectively

contribute to the dynamic interplay
influencing the metabolic landscape.

CHAPTER 3

The Science Behind the Metabolic Flexibility Diet

3.1 Cellular Energy Production

At the heart of metabolic flexibility lies the awe-inspiring process of cellular energy production, intricately woven through a series of biochemical pathways within the confines of our cells. Central to this process is the mitochondrion, an organelle often referred to as the powerhouse of the cell.

The journey begins with the catabolism of macronutrients, a fundamental process that breaks down carbohydrates, fats, and proteins into their constituent parts.

Glucose, derived from carbohydrates, enters glycolysis, a sequence of enzymatic reactions that yield pyruvate. Meanwhile, fatty acids are broken down through beta-oxidation, producing acetyl-CoA. Simultaneously, proteins are cleaved into amino acids, some of which can be converted into intermediates entering the same energy-producing pathways.

The pivotal point converges at the citric acid cycle, where both pyruvate and acetyl-CoA contribute to a series of chemical reactions, ultimately generating reducing equivalents in the form of NADH and FADH2. These electron carriers become critical as they fuel the electron transport chain, an intricate molecular machinery embedded in the inner mitochondrial membrane.

As electrons travel through the electron transport chain, a flow akin to a cascade is established. This sets the stage for the pumping of protons across the mitochondrial membrane, creating an electrochemical gradient. The culmination of this process occurs as protons flow back into the mitochondrial matrix through ATP synthase, driving the synthesis of ATP from adenosine diphosphate (ADP) and inorganic phosphate.

This orchestrated dance of molecules—acetyl-CoA, NADH, FADH2, and ATP—defines the cellular ballet of energy production. The section not only elucidates the elegance of these processes but also underscores the significance of their adaptability. The ability of the cell to flexibly switch between utilizing glucose and fatty acids for energy production stands as a testament to the body's inherent capacity for metabolic adaptability.

Understanding the intricacies of cellular energy production lays a foundation for the subsequent exploration of how dietary and lifestyle choices can

modulate these pathways, fostering a
metabolic milieu conducive to flexibility.
As we unravel the molecular ballet
within our cells, the Metabolic
Flexibility Diet begins to emerge not
merely as a dietary approach but as a
harmonious orchestration of nutrition,
physiology, and cellular dynamics.

3.2 Hormonal Regulation

In the symphony of metabolic flexibility,
hormones emerge as the conductors,
orchestrating the intricate balance
between energy storage and expenditure.
We will delves into the profound
influence of hormones on metabolic
regulation, shedding light on how these
molecular messengers harmonize the
cellular dance of energy metabolism.

At the forefront is insulin, a hormone
produced by the pancreas in response to
elevated blood glucose levels. Insulin
acts as a key player in facilitating the

uptake of glucose by cells, promoting its conversion into glycogen for storage in the liver and muscles. Simultaneously, insulin inhibits the breakdown of stored fats, directing the body towards utilizing glucose as a primary energy source.

Contrastingly, glucagon, insulin's counterpart, rises in response to low blood glucose levels. It prompts the liver to break down glycogen into glucose, releasing it into the bloodstream. Moreover, glucagon stimulates the breakdown of fats into fatty acids, fostering their utilization as an alternative energy substrate.

The delicate interplay between insulin and glucagon, often referred to as the insulin-glucagon axis, exemplifies the hormonal regulation intrinsic to metabolic flexibility. Furthermore, hormones such as cortisol, adrenaline, and growth hormone intricately modulate metabolism in response to various stressors and stimuli, further sculpting the body's adaptive capacity.

Beyond the classic players, emerging hormones such as adiponectin and leptin, secreted by adipose tissue, exert profound effects on metabolic flexibility. Adiponectin enhances insulin sensitivity, promoting efficient glucose utilization, while leptin communicates satiety signals to the brain, influencing food intake and energy expenditure.

3.3 Nutrient Utilization

In the intricate dance of metabolic flexibility, nutrient utilization emerges as a dynamic process, finely tuned to the body's ever-changing energy demands.

Carbohydrates, as a primary energy source, undergo glycolysis, a series of enzymatic reactions that yield pyruvate. This pyruvate can then be directed towards aerobic metabolism, producing

ATP in the presence of oxygen, or anaerobic metabolism, generating lactate in the absence of oxygen.

Fats, stored in adipose tissue, are mobilized through lipolysis, breaking down triglycerides into glycerol and fatty acids. The fatty acids, in turn, undergo beta-oxidation within the mitochondria, yielding acetyl-CoA—a key player in the citric acid cycle. The ability of the body to efficiently switch between glucose and fatty acids as energy substrates epitomizes metabolic flexibility.

Proteins, although not the primary energy source, contribute amino acids that can enter the citric acid cycle or be converted into glucose through gluconeogenesis. This adaptability underscores the body's capacity to derive energy from diverse nutrient sources, ensuring a constant supply even in the absence of a specific macronutrient.

CHAPTER 4

Principles of the Metabolic Flexibility Diet

4.1 Balanced Macronutrient Ratios

As we venture into the core principles of the Metabolic Flexibility Diet, the first pillar we encounter is the delicate balance of macronutrients. We will delve into the significance of maintaining optimal ratios of carbohydrates, fats, and proteins to foster a metabolic environment that embraces flexibility and efficiency.

At the heart of metabolic flexibility lies the art of crafting a diet that harmonizes the trio of macronutrients—

carbohydrates, fats, and proteins. The delicate interplay between these essential components becomes the cornerstone of the Metabolic Flexibility Diet, reflecting a recognition of the body's adaptive capacity to utilize different energy sources.

- *Carbohydrates:* Often vilified in some dietary narratives, carbohydrates are, in fact, a fundamental player in the metabolic symphony. The key lies in the type and quality of carbohydrates consumed. Emphasizing complex carbohydrates such as whole grains, legumes, and vegetables provides a sustained release of glucose, avoiding the blood sugar rollercoaster associated with refined sugars. This not only supports stable energy levels but also facilitates the body's ability to switch between glucose and fats as primary energy sources.

- *Fats:* Healthy fats, including monounsaturated and polyunsaturated fats, take center stage in promoting metabolic flexibility. These fats, found in sources like avocados, nuts, seeds, and fatty fish, contribute to cellular integrity and serve as a valuable reservoir of energy. Striking a balance between omega-3 and omega-6 fatty acids further fine-tunes the inflammatory response, a key player in metabolic health.

- *Proteins:* Beyond their role in muscle building, proteins contribute to satiety and play a crucial role in the metabolic flexibility dance. Diversifying protein sources to include lean meats, poultry, fish, eggs, legumes, and plant-based options ensures a spectrum of amino acids, supporting both energy production and tissue repair.

The Metabolic Flexibility Diet emphasizes the adaptability of macronutrient ratios, acknowledging that individual needs may vary based on factors such as activity levels, metabolic rate, and health goals. While some individuals may thrive with a slightly higher intake of carbohydrates, others may find greater benefit in a diet richer in fats. The key lies in personalization and a holistic approach that considers the unique metabolic fingerprint of each individual.

By implementing balanced macronutrient ratios, the Metabolic Flexibility Diet becomes a flexible framework that not only adapts to individual needs but also nourishes the body with the diverse array of nutrients essential for optimal metabolic function. This principle lays the foundation for the subsequent exploration of meal timing and other lifestyle factors within the Metabolic Flexibility Diet.

4.2 Timing of Meals

The rhythmic cadence of meal timing holds profound implications for metabolic flexibility, as the body's circadian rhythms intricately intertwine with nutritional cues. Understanding the temporal aspects of nourishment allows for a strategic alignment of eating patterns with the body's natural rhythms, optimizing metabolic processes.

- *Breakfast as a Metabolic Ignition:* Breakfast, often hailed as the "most important meal of the day," serves as a metabolic ignition switch. By breaking the overnight fast, breakfast kickstarts the metabolism, signaling to the body that a new day of energy expenditure has begun. A balanced breakfast, rich in protein and complex carbohydrates, sets the stage for stable blood sugar levels and sustained energy throughout the day.

- *Strategic Nutrient Timing:* Beyond the conventional three meals a day, the Metabolic Flexibility Diet embraces a nuanced approach to nutrient timing. Incorporating snacks strategically between meals, particularly when facing prolonged gaps, helps maintain stable blood glucose levels. This practice prevents excessive hunger, reducing the likelihood of overconsumption during main meals and supporting the body's ability to efficiently utilize nutrients.

- *Evening Considerations:* Recognizing the body's evolving needs throughout the day, the composition of evening meals takes center stage. A focus on lean proteins, fiber-rich vegetables, and healthy fats supports satiety and minimizes the risk of blood sugar fluctuations during the night. Additionally, allowing an interval between the last meal and bedtime aligns with the body's natural fasting period during sleep, fostering metabolic adaptability.

- *Intermittent Fasting as a Tool:* Intermittent fasting, a temporal approach to eating, has gained traction for its potential to enhance metabolic flexibility. By incorporating periods of fasting, the body is prompted to tap into stored energy reserves, promoting the efficient utilization of both glucose and fats. This practice aligns with the body's inherent fasting and feeding cycles, fostering resilience and adaptability.

meal timing within the Metabolic Flexibility Diet transcends rigid schedules; it involves attunement to the body's cues and natural rhythms. This principle emphasizes the dynamic nature of metabolism, highlighting that when we eat is as crucial as what we eat. By aligning nourishment with the body's temporal rhythms, the Metabolic Flexibility Diet unfolds as a holistic approach that transcends mere caloric considerations, embracing the intricate dance between nutrition and circadian biology.

4.3 Impact of Exercise on Metabolic Flexibility

Exercise stands as a cornerstone in the architecture of metabolic flexibility, acting as a potent modulator of cellular processes that govern energy metabolism. The dynamic interplay between physical activity and the intricate pathways of metabolism orchestrates a cascade of physiological adaptations that extend far beyond the realms of calorie expenditure.

- *Aerobic Exercise and Mitochondrial Biogenesis:* Aerobic exercise, characterized by sustained and rhythmic activities such as running, swimming, or cycling, emerges as a catalyst for mitochondrial biogenesis. Mitochondria, the cellular powerhouses, undergo proliferation in response to the increased energy demand posed by aerobic activities. This not only enhances the capacity for aerobic metabolism but also fortifies the cellular foundation for metabolic flexibility.

- *Resistance Training and Muscle Metabolism:* Resistance training, encompassing activities like weightlifting and bodyweight exercises, exerts a profound influence on muscle metabolism. The hypertrophy and strengthening of muscle tissue not only contribute to overall metabolic rate but also enhance the capacity of muscles to store and utilize glycogen—a crucial substrate for energy production.

- *High-Intensity Interval Training (HIIT) and Metabolic Adaptations:* HIIT, characterized by short bursts of intense activity interspersed with periods of rest or lower-intensity exercise, induces rapid metabolic adaptations. This form of exercise enhances both aerobic and anaerobic capacities, promoting the efficient utilization of both carbohydrates and fats for energy. The "afterburn" effect, known as excess post-exercise oxygen consumption (EPOC), further extends the metabolic benefits beyond the workout session.

- *Timing and Type of Exercise:* The temporal dimension of exercise, much like meal timing, plays a role in optimizing metabolic flexibility. Morning exercise, for instance, aligns with the body's natural cortisol rhythm, potentially enhancing fat oxidation. Furthermore, incorporating a mix of aerobic and resistance exercises ensures a comprehensive approach, addressing various facets of metabolic health.

The impact of exercise on metabolic flexibility extends beyond calorie burning; it encompasses a nuanced orchestration of cellular responses that fine-tune the body's ability to adapt to different energy demands. The Metabolic Flexibility Diet, therefore, integrates physical activity as an integral component, recognizing its role not only in weight management but also in sculpting a resilient and adaptable metabolism.

CHAPTER 5

Key Components of the Metabolic Flexibility Diet

5.1 High-Quality Protein Sources

Transitioning from principles to actionable components, the Metabolic Flexibility Diet unveils a series of key elements that lay the groundwork for a resilient and adaptive metabolism. Among these components, the quality and strategic incorporation of protein sources take center stage, shaping the dietary landscape to optimize metabolic flexibility.

Protein, often heralded as the building block of life, assumes a pivotal role in the Metabolic Flexibility Diet. Beyond its muscle-building reputation, the quality and diversity of protein sources become essential factors influencing metabolic adaptability.

- *Lean Animal Proteins:* Incorporating lean animal proteins, such as poultry, fish, and lean cuts of meat, provides a spectrum of essential amino acids crucial for cellular function and repair. These proteins not only support muscle maintenance but also contribute to the thermic effect of food, enhancing overall energy expenditure.

- *Plant-Based Proteins:* Diversifying protein sources to include plant-based options contributes to the metabolic flexibility tapestry. Legumes, lentils, beans, tofu, and tempeh offer not only protein but also fiber and micronutrients that synergistically support metabolic health. This plant-centric approach aligns with evidence suggesting that plant-based diets may confer metabolic benefits.

- *Omega-3 Rich Foods:* Fatty fish, such as salmon, mackerel, and sardines, not only serve as excellent sources of protein but also provide omega-3 fatty acids. These essential fats play a role in reducing inflammation and promoting metabolic flexibility by influencing cellular membrane composition and function.

- *Dairy and Eggs:* Dairy products, including Greek yogurt and cottage cheese, offer protein along with calcium and probiotics. Eggs, rich in high-quality proteins and various nutrients, contribute to satiety and support metabolic function. The inclusion of these dairy and egg-based proteins enhances dietary variety and nutrient density.

- *Protein Timing:* The strategic distribution of protein throughout the day becomes a key consideration in optimizing metabolic flexibility. Incorporating protein into each meal and snack not only supports satiety but also promotes the maintenance of lean body mass— a critical factor in sustaining a robust metabolism.

By prioritizing high-quality protein sources, the Metabolic Flexibility Diet emphasizes the importance of a diverse and nutrient-dense approach to nourishment. The nuanced selection of proteins not only fulfills the body's structural and functional needs but also supports the intricate dance of cellular processes that govern metabolic adaptability. As we delve into the key components of this diet, the spotlight on protein underscores its central role in sculpting a metabolism that is not only flexible but also resilient and primed for optimal function.

5.2 Healthy Fats for Metabolic Health

Dispelling the antiquated notion that all fats are created equal, the Metabolic Flexibility Diet champions the inclusion of healthy fats, recognizing their diverse roles in cellular function, hormone regulation, and energy metabolism.

- *Monounsaturated Fats:* Abundant in sources such as olive oil, avocados, and nuts, monounsaturated fats contribute to metabolic flexibility by promoting insulin sensitivity. These fats not only provide a rich source of energy but also confer anti-inflammatory properties, supporting overall metabolic health.

- *Polyunsaturated Fats:* Omega-3 and omega-6 fatty acids, classified as polyunsaturated fats, play a pivotal role in the Metabolic Flexibility Diet. Fatty fish, flaxseeds, chia seeds, and walnuts are rich sources of omega-3s, known for their anti-inflammatory effects and potential to enhance insulin sensitivity. Striking a balance between omega-3s and omega-6s supports a harmonious inflammatory response, a key aspect of metabolic resilience.

- *Saturated Fats in Moderation:* While the diet acknowledges the role of saturated fats in cellular structure and hormone production, moderation remains key.

Incorporating sources like coconut oil, dairy, and lean cuts of meat adds flavor and variety without compromising metabolic health. Strategic selection and mindful portions ensure a balanced intake.

- *Medium-Chain Triglycerides (MCTs):* Found in coconut oil and certain dairy products, MCTs are a unique form of saturated fat with potential metabolic benefits. They are rapidly absorbed and metabolized, offering a quick source of energy. Including MCTs in the diet may support ketone production, especially relevant for individuals exploring low-carbohydrate or ketogenic approaches.

- *Avoidance of Trans Fats:* The Metabolic Flexibility Diet emphatically discourages the consumption of trans fats—

artificially hydrogenated fats found in many processed foods. These fats not only contribute to inflammation but also interfere with cellular function, undermining metabolic flexibility.

Promoting a judicious selection of healthy fats, the Metabolic Flexibility Diet harnesses the diverse benefits of fats while mitigating potential risks. This approach not only satiates the palate but also nourishes the body at the cellular level, fortifying the foundation for metabolic adaptability. As we weave through the key components of this diet, the emphasis on healthy fats emerges as a pivotal element in sculpting a diet that embraces flexibility, resilience, and sustained metabolic health.

5.3 Carbohydrates: Types and Timing

In the intricate tapestry of the Metabolic Flexibility Diet, the role of carbohydrates emerges as a critical determinant of metabolic health.

Carbohydrates, often at the center of dietary debates, assume a nuanced role in the Metabolic Flexibility Diet. Recognizing the diversity of carbohydrates and the temporal dimension of their consumption becomes pivotal in shaping a diet that harmonizes with the body's innate capacity for metabolic adaptability.

- *Complex Carbohydrates for Sustained Energy:* The diet prioritizes complex carbohydrates derived from whole, unprocessed sources such as whole grains, legumes, and vegetables. These carbohydrates, rich in fiber and nutrients, facilitate a gradual release of glucose into the bloodstream, supporting stable energy levels and minimizing the risk of abrupt blood sugar spikes and crashes.

- *Fruits for Natural Sugars and Fiber:* While fruits contribute natural sugars, they are accompanied by fiber, vitamins, and antioxidants. The inclusion of a variety of fruits aligns with the diet's emphasis on nutrient density, ensuring that carbohydrates are not only a source of energy but also a vehicle for essential micronutrients.

- *Strategic Carbohydrate Timing:* The temporal distribution of carbohydrates throughout the day becomes a strategic consideration. The Metabolic Flexibility Diet encourages a higher carbohydrate intake during periods of increased energy demand, such as around workouts. This practice optimizes the utilization of glucose for energy, minimizing the likelihood of excess glucose being stored as fat.

- *Cyclic Carbohydrate Periodization:* Some iterations of the Metabolic Flexibility Diet incorporate cyclic carbohydrate periodization. This approach involves alternating between higher and lower carbohydrate days, promoting the body's ability to switch between fuel sources. It mimics the natural ebb and flow of carbohydrate availability in the environment, encouraging metabolic flexibility.

- *Mindful Selection of Carbohydrate Sources:* The diet advocates for a discerning approach to carbohydrate sources, steering away from refined sugars and processed grains. Instead, it encourages the consumption of nutrient-dense carbohydrates that contribute not only to energy needs but also to overall well-being.

The Metabolic Flexibility Diet views carbohydrates not as adversaries but as dynamic contributors to the body's energy orchestra. By selecting the right types of carbohydrates and strategically timing their consumption, this diet capitalizes on the inherent adaptability of the metabolism.

CHAPTER 6

Meal Planning for Metabolic Flexibility

6.1 Sample Meal Plans

- **Day 1: Balanced Macronutrient Day**

  - *Breakfast:* Scrambled eggs with spinach and tomatoes, whole-grain toast.

  - *Mid-Morning Snack:* Greek yogurt with mixed berries and a sprinkle of chia seeds.

  - *Lunch:* Grilled chicken salad with a variety of colorful vegetables, quinoa, and a vinaigrette dressing.

- *Afternoon Snack:* Handful
  of almonds with an apple.

- *Dinner:* Baked salmon
  with sweet potato wedges
  and steamed broccoli.

- **Day 2: Carbohydrate Cycling
  Day**

  - *Breakfast:* Oatmeal with
    sliced banana and a
    teaspoon of almond butter.

  - *Mid-Morning Snack:*
    Cottage cheese with
    pineapple chunks.

  - *Lunch:* Lentil soup with a
    side of mixed greens.

  - *Afternoon Snack:* Carrot
    and cucumber sticks with
    hummus.

  - *Dinner:* Grilled shrimp
    with quinoa and roasted
    Brussels sprouts.

- **Day 3: Intermittent Fasting Day**

  - *Morning (During Fasting Period):* Black coffee, herbal tea, or water.

  - *Breakfast (Breaking Fast):* Scrambled eggs with avocado and whole-grain toast.

  - *Mid-Morning Snack:* Green smoothie with spinach, banana, and protein powder.

  - *Lunch:* Chicken and vegetable stir-fry with brown rice.

  - *Afternoon Snack:* Handful of walnuts with a small apple.

  - *Dinner:* Baked cod with roasted sweet potatoes and asparagus.

- **Day 4: High-Intensity Interval Training (HIIT) Day**

  - *Pre-Workout Snack:* Whole-grain toast with almond butter.

  - *Post-Workout Meal:* Protein smoothie with whey protein, banana, and a handful of berries.

  - *Lunch:* Quinoa salad with mixed vegetables and grilled chicken.

  - *Afternoon Snack:* Greek yogurt with a drizzle of honey.

  - *Dinner:* Turkey meatballs with zucchini noodles and tomato sauce.

- **Day 5: Plant-Centric Day**

- *Breakfast:* Smoothie bowl with kale, pineapple, and chia seeds.

- *Mid-Morning Snack:* Handful of mixed nuts.

- *Lunch:* Chickpea and vegetable curry with brown rice.

- *Afternoon Snack:* Sliced cucumber and cherry tomatoes with guacamole.

- *Dinner:* Stir-fried tofu with broccoli, bell peppers, and quinoa.

These sample meal plans showcase the flexibility and diversity inherent in the Metabolic Flexibility Diet. The emphasis on nutrient-dense foods, balanced macronutrient ratios, and strategic meal timing aligns with the principles of metabolic adaptability. These plans serve as a template, with room for customization based on individual preferences, dietary needs, and activity levels. As one journeys through the Metabolic Flexibility Diet, these meal plans provide a practical guide for translating principles into actionable and delicious meals that support a resilient and adaptable metabolism.

6.2 Adapting the Diet to Personal Needs

The Metabolic Flexibility Diet, while providing a structured framework, is inherently adaptable to individual needs, preferences, and goals.

1. **Caloric Requirements:** The Metabolic Flexibility Diet is not a one-size-fits-all approach. Individuals with different caloric needs due to variations in age, gender, activity levels, and metabolism should adjust portion

sizes accordingly. Understanding one's caloric requirements is crucial for maintaining a balance between energy intake and expenditure.

2. **Macronutrient Ratios:** The ideal macronutrient distribution may vary based on individual factors such as metabolic rate, fitness goals, and dietary preferences. Some individuals may thrive on a slightly higher carbohydrate intake, while others may benefit from a more ketogenic approach. Experimenting with macronutrient ratios allows for personalization.

3. **Meal Timing and Frequency:** The temporal aspect of meal timing can be personalized to align with individual lifestyles and preferences. While some individuals may find benefit in intermittent fasting, others may prefer a more traditional three-

meals-a-day structure. Adapting meal timing to accommodate workouts or personal schedules enhances sustainability.

4. **Food Sensitivities and Allergies:** Consideration of individual sensitivities and allergies is paramount. The Metabolic Flexibility Diet encourages the selection of nutrient-dense whole foods, but it's crucial to avoid items that may trigger adverse reactions. Substituting ingredients while maintaining the principles of the diet ensures a tailored approach.

5. **Fitness Goals:** Individuals with specific fitness goals, such as muscle gain or fat loss, can adjust the diet to support these objectives. Fine-tuning macronutrient ratios, caloric intake, and meal timing aligns nutrition with fitness aspirations,

optimizing the diet's impact on body composition and performance.

6. **Health Conditions:** Individuals with specific health conditions, such as diabetes, cardiovascular issues, or metabolic disorders, should collaborate with healthcare professionals to adapt the diet appropriately. Customizing carbohydrate intake, selecting heart-healthy fats, and monitoring blood sugar levels are examples of adjustments based on health considerations.

7. **Cultural and Dietary Preferences:** The Metabolic Flexibility Diet is versatile and can be adapted to various cultural and dietary preferences. Substituting ingredients or modifying recipes to align with personal tastes ensures that the

diet is not only effective but also enjoyable and sustainable.

8. **Monitoring and Adjusting:** Regular monitoring of progress and listening to one's body are essential components of adapting the diet. Adjustments may be necessary based on how the body responds to dietary changes, energy levels, and overall well-being. Flexibility and openness to modification contribute to long-term success.

Adapting the Metabolic Flexibility Diet to personal needs involves a balance between the foundational principles and individual variations. experimenting with different approaches allows for the discovery of an optimal and sustainable dietary strategy that fosters metabolic adaptability while aligning with personal preferences and goals.

CHAPTER 7

Supplements and Metabolic Flexibility

7.1 Essential Nutrients

Supplements can play a supportive role in enhancing metabolic flexibility, especially when there are specific nutrient gaps or lifestyle factors that may impact optimal nutrition.

While the Metabolic Flexibility Diet emphasizes obtaining nutrients from whole foods, there are situations where supplementation may be beneficial to address specific needs. Here are key essential nutrients to consider:

1. **Omega-3 Fatty Acids:** Supplementing with omega-3 fatty acids, particularly EPA (eicosapentaenoic acid) and DHA

(docosahexaenoic acid), can support cardiovascular health, reduce inflammation, and contribute to optimal brain function. Fish oil supplements or algae-based supplements are common sources.

2. **Vitamin D:** Many individuals may have inadequate vitamin D levels, especially if they have limited sun exposure. Vitamin D is crucial for bone health, immune function, and may play a role in metabolic regulation. Supplementation can be considered, especially in regions with limited sunlight.

3. **Magnesium:** Magnesium is involved in numerous enzymatic reactions, including those related to energy metabolism. It plays a role in insulin sensitivity and glucose regulation. Supplementation may be

considered for individuals with low dietary intake or those experiencing symptoms of magnesium deficiency.

4. **B Vitamins:** B vitamins, including B6, B12, and folate, play essential roles in energy metabolism and the synthesis of neurotransmitters. Supplementing with B vitamins may be beneficial for individuals with specific dietary restrictions, such as vegetarians and vegans, or those with impaired absorption.

5. **Protein Supplements:** In certain situations, such as intense physical training or difficulty meeting protein needs through whole foods, protein supplements like whey or plant-based protein powders can support muscle maintenance and recovery.

6. **Electrolytes:** For individuals engaged in strenuous physical activity or following a low-carbohydrate diet, supplementing with electrolytes (sodium, potassium, magnesium) can help maintain fluid balance, support muscle function, and prevent dehydration.

7. **Probiotics:** Gut health is linked to metabolic health, and probiotics can contribute to a healthy gut microbiome. Probiotic supplements may be considered, especially after antibiotic use or for individuals with digestive issues.

8. **Coenzyme Q10 (CoQ10):** CoQ10 is involved in cellular energy production and has antioxidant properties. Supplementation may be beneficial for individuals with certain medical conditions or

those on medications that deplete CoQ10.

It's crucial to note that while supplements can fill nutrient gaps, they are not a substitute for a well-rounded diet. Individual needs vary, and consulting with a healthcare professional before initiating any supplementation is recommended. Regular monitoring and adjustments to supplement regimens based on changing health status or dietary patterns contribute to a holistic approach to metabolic flexibility.

7.2 Supplements that Support Metabolic Health

In the pursuit of metabolic flexibility, certain supplements can be strategically chosen to support overall metabolic health and optimize the body's ability to adapt to different energy sources.

1. **Alpha-Lipoic Acid (ALA):** ALA is an antioxidant that has been studied for its potential benefits in improving insulin sensitivity. It may assist in glucose uptake and utilization, contributing to better metabolic flexibility.

2. **Berberine:** Berberine is a compound extracted from several plants and has been shown to have glucose-lowering effects. It may help regulate blood sugar levels and enhance insulin sensitivity, promoting metabolic adaptability.

3. **Cinnamon:** Cinnamon supplementation has been associated with improved insulin sensitivity and may contribute to better glycemic control. Including cinnamon as a spice or taking it in supplement form can be a flavorful addition to support metabolic health.

4. **Chromium:** Chromium is a trace mineral that plays a role in insulin signaling. Supplementing with chromium may support insulin sensitivity and glucose metabolism, promoting a more flexible response to dietary carbohydrates.

5. **Green Tea Extract:** Green tea contains catechins, compounds with antioxidant properties. Green tea extract supplementation has been linked to improved fat oxidation and may contribute to metabolic flexibility by enhancing the body's ability to use fats for energy.

6. **Resveratrol:** Found in red wine and certain foods, resveratrol is a polyphenol with antioxidant properties. It has been studied for its potential to improve insulin sensitivity and support metabolic health.

7. **L-Carnitine:** L-Carnitine is involved in the transport of fatty acids into the mitochondria, where they are used for energy production. Supplementing with L-Carnitine may support the efficient utilization of fats as an energy source.

8. **Curcumin (Turmeric):** Curcumin, the active compound in turmeric, has anti-inflammatory and antioxidant properties. It may contribute to metabolic flexibility by modulating inflammatory pathways and supporting overall metabolic health.

9. **Vitamin K2:** Vitamin K2 plays a role in calcium metabolism and has been associated with improved insulin sensitivity. Including vitamin K2-rich foods or considering supplementation may be beneficial for metabolic health.

10. **N-Acetyl Cysteine (NAC):** NAC is a precursor to glutathione, a powerful antioxidant. It may have potential benefits in improving insulin sensitivity and reducing oxidative stress, contributing to metabolic resilience.

While these supplements show promise in supporting metabolic health, it's essential to approach supplementation with caution and individualization. Consulting with a healthcare professional before adding supplements to your routine is advised, as individual responses may vary, and excessive supplementation can have unintended consequences. Additionally, focusing on a nutrient-dense diet and lifestyle factors remains foundational for achieving and maintaining metabolic flexibility.

CHAPTER 8

Lifestyle Factors and Metabolic Flexibility

In the intricate dance of metabolic flexibility, lifestyle factors play a pivotal role in shaping the body's ability to adapt to varying energy demands.

8.1 Importance of Sleep

Quality sleep is the unsung hero of metabolic flexibility. The intricate web of hormonal regulation, cellular repair, and energy metabolism is finely tuned during the restorative hours of sleep. Here's why prioritizing quality sleep is crucial for optimal metabolic function:

1. **Hormonal Harmony:** Sleep duration and quality influence

hormones such as leptin and ghrelin, which regulate hunger and satiety. Inadequate sleep can disrupt this delicate balance, leading to increased appetite and potential overconsumption of calories.

2. **Insulin Sensitivity:** Lack of sleep has been linked to reduced insulin sensitivity, akin to the effects of insulin resistance. This can impair the body's ability to efficiently utilize glucose, potentially contributing to metabolic inflexibility.

3. **Cortisol Regulation:** Sleep deprivation can elevate cortisol levels, the body's primary stress hormone. Elevated cortisol is associated with insulin resistance and an increased likelihood of storing energy as abdominal fat.

4. **Energy Expenditure:** Quality sleep contributes to overall energy expenditure. Adequate rest supports physical recovery, sustains mental focus, and enhances the body's capacity to engage in regular physical activity—an integral component of metabolic flexibility.

Tips for Improving Sleep:

- Maintain a consistent sleep schedule.

- Create a conducive sleep environment (cool, dark, and quiet).

- Limit screen time before bedtime.

- Practice relaxation techniques, such as deep breathing or meditation.

8.2 Stress Management

Stress, whether physical or psychological, can tip the delicate balance of metabolic flexibility. Chronic stress prompts a cascade of hormonal responses that can impact energy metabolism and contribute to metabolic dysfunction. Here's why effective stress management is pivotal:

1. **Cortisol Dynamics:** Chronic stress can lead to dysregulation of cortisol, disrupting its natural rhythm. Elevated cortisol levels are associated with increased abdominal fat deposition and impaired insulin sensitivity.

2. **Inflammation:** Stress induces inflammation, a factor intricately linked to metabolic disorders. Chronic low-grade inflammation can impede the body's ability to switch between energy sources,

compromising metabolic flexibility.

3. **Food Choices and Cravings:** Stress often influences food choices, with a tendency to opt for comfort foods high in sugar and fats. These dietary choices can further impact metabolic health and contribute to insulin resistance.

4. **Physical Activity:** While exercise is a key component of metabolic flexibility, excessive and intense physical activity without adequate recovery can become a stressor. Balancing exercise with restorative practices is essential for optimizing metabolic health.

Tips for Effective Stress Management:

- Incorporate relaxation techniques (meditation, yoga, deep breathing).

- Prioritize leisure activities and hobbies.

- Foster a supportive social network.

- Ensure adequate downtime and restorative sleep.

By acknowledging the interplay between lifestyle factors and metabolic flexibility, individuals can empower themselves to make holistic choices that support not only optimal metabolic health but also overall well-being. The Metabolic Flexibility Diet, when complemented by sound lifestyle practices, becomes a comprehensive approach to cultivating a resilient and adaptable metabolism.

CHAPTER 9

Common Challenges and Solutions

9.1 Overcoming Plateaus

In the journey toward metabolic flexibility, individuals may encounter various challenges that can impede progress. One common hurdle is the experience of plateaus, where noticeable improvements in metabolic health and flexibility seem to stall.

Plateaus are a natural part of any transformative journey, and understanding how to navigate them is key to sustained progress. Here are strategies to overcome plateaus in the pursuit of metabolic flexibility:

1. **Reassess Nutrient Intake:** As the body adapts to dietary changes,

metabolic needs may evolve.
Reevaluate your caloric intake,
macronutrient ratios, and overall
nutrient balance. Adjusting
portion sizes or tweaking
macronutrient distribution can
reignite progress.

2. **Introduce Variety:** The body
responds positively to variety. If
your diet has become too routine,
introduce new foods, recipes, and
flavors. This not only enhances
nutritional diversity but also
prevents metabolic adaptation to a
consistent dietary pattern.

3. **Modify Exercise Routine:**
Plateaus can also manifest in
exercise adaptations. Assess your
workout routine and consider
introducing new exercises,
varying intensity, or incorporating
different forms of physical
activity. This challenges the body,
promoting continued adaptation.

4. **Implement Fasting Strategies:**
    Intermittent fasting or modified
    fasting approaches can be
    effective in breaking plateaus.
    Periods of fasting prompt the
    body to tap into stored energy
    reserves, fostering metabolic
    flexibility.

5. **Evaluate Sleep Quality:**
    Insufficient or poor-quality sleep
    can hinder metabolic progress.
    Reassess your sleep habits and
    prioritize strategies to improve
    sleep hygiene. Quality rest
    supports overall well-being and
    metabolic resilience.

6. **Manage Stress Levels:** Chronic
    stress can contribute to plateaus
    by influencing hormonal balance.
    Incorporate stress management
    techniques, such as meditation,
    deep breathing, or relaxation
    exercises, to support metabolic
    health.

7. **Consider Refeed Days:**
    Introducing occasional refeed days with a temporary increase in caloric intake, especially from carbohydrates, can signal to the body that resources are plentiful. This can help overcome metabolic adaptations associated with prolonged caloric restriction.

8. **Monitor Non-Scale Metrics:**
    Shift the focus from solely relying on the scale. Track non-scale metrics like energy levels, sleep quality, mood, and physical performance. Positive changes in these areas indicate progress beyond mere weight loss.

9. **Consult a Professional:** If plateaus persist, consider consulting with a nutritionist, dietitian, or healthcare professional. They can provide personalized guidance, identify potential barriers, and offer

targeted solutions based on your
individual needs.

10. **Patience and Consistency:**
Transformation takes time.
Plateaus are a natural part of the
process, and perseverance is key.
Stay consistent with your dietary
and lifestyle changes, recognizing
that long-term improvements
often involve gradual, sustainable
shifts.

approaching plateaus with a combination
of strategic adjustments and a holistic
perspective, individuals can navigate
these challenges on the path to enhanced
metabolic flexibility. The Metabolic
Flexibility Diet, when dynamically
adapted to individual needs, remains a
powerful tool for achieving and
maintaining optimal metabolic health.

9.2 Dealing with Cravings

Cravings can be a formidable obstacle on the path to metabolic flexibility, but understanding their origins and implementing targeted strategies can empower individuals to overcome them.

1. **Identify Triggers:** Recognize the specific triggers that lead to cravings. Whether they are emotional, environmental, or tied to specific foods, understanding the root cause is the first step in managing cravings.

2. **Balanced Meals:** Ensure that meals are well-balanced, incorporating a mix of protein, healthy fats, and complex carbohydrates. Balanced meals provide sustained energy and help prevent sudden blood sugar fluctuations that can trigger cravings.

3. **Hydration:** Dehydration can sometimes masquerade as hunger or cravings. Stay adequately hydrated throughout the day, as water intake can help manage appetite and reduce the intensity of cravings.

4. **Satisfying Alternatives:** Identify healthier alternatives to satisfy cravings. For example, if you crave something sweet, opt for a piece of fruit or a small serving of dark chocolate. Finding nutritious substitutes can help meet cravings without derailing progress.

5. **Mindful Eating:** Practice mindful eating by paying attention to the sensory aspects of each bite. Engage all your senses, savor the flavors, and eat slowly. This can enhance satisfaction and reduce the intensity of cravings.

6. **Strategic Indulgences:** Allow yourself occasional indulgences in a controlled and mindful manner. Completely restricting certain foods may intensify cravings. Allowing small treats can contribute to a balanced and sustainable approach.

7. **Manage Stress:** Stress is a common trigger for cravings, especially for comfort foods. Implement stress management techniques such as deep breathing, meditation, or physical activity to reduce stress levels.

8. **Sleep Quality:** Ensure you are getting sufficient and quality sleep. Inadequate sleep can disrupt hormonal balance, increasing the likelihood of cravings. Prioritize rest to support overall metabolic health.

9. **Protein Intake:** Include an adequate amount of protein in your meals and snacks. Protein has a satiating effect, helping to curb hunger and reduce the likelihood of experiencing intense cravings.

10. **Plan Ahead:** Plan meals and snacks in advance to avoid situations where you might be tempted by unhealthy food choices. Having nutritious options readily available can help prevent impulsive choices driven by cravings.

9.3 Social and Practical Considerations

Social and practical considerations are integral aspects of a sustainable approach to metabolic flexibility. Balancing dietary choices with social interactions and daily routines enhances the feasibility and enjoyment of the Metabolic Flexibility Diet.

1. **Communicate Dietary Preferences:** Clearly communicate your dietary preferences and goals to friends and family. This foster understanding and support, reducing potential social pressure to deviate from your chosen dietary approach.

2. **Flexible Choices in Social Settings:** When dining out or attending social events, aim for flexibility. Choose options that align with the principles of the Metabolic Flexibility Diet while allowing for some degree of variety and enjoyment.

3. **Bring Your Own Dish:** If feasible, contribute a dish to social gatherings. This ensures

that there is at least one option that aligns with your dietary preferences, and it can be a positive way to share your approach with others.

4. **Plan Ahead for Travel:** When traveling, plan ahead by researching food options at your destination. Pack nutritious snacks, and consider bringing portable meal options to maintain consistency with your dietary goals.

5. **Educate Others:** Take the opportunity to educate friends and family about the Metabolic Flexibility Diet. Share information about the benefits and rationale behind your choices, fostering a supportive environment.

6. **Stay Mindful of Portions:** In social settings, be mindful of

portion sizes. It's possible to enjoy a variety of foods while still adhering to the principles of the diet. Portion control is a key factor in maintaining balance.

7. **Be Adaptable:** Embrace adaptability in your approach. Life is dynamic, and situations may arise that necessitate flexibility in your dietary choices. Being adaptable while staying true to the core principles ensures long-term sustainability.

8. **Incorporate Social Activities:** Plan social activities that don't solely revolve around food. Engaging in physical activities, cultural events, or recreational pursuits provides alternative avenues for social interactions.

Proactively addressing cravings and navigating social and practical considerations, individuals can foster a balanced and sustainable approach to the Metabolic Flexibility Diet. Recognizing these challenges as integral components of the journey allows for strategic planning and a resilient mindset on the path to optimal metabolic health.

9.4 Looking Ahead on Your Metabolic Flexibility Journey

As you continue your journey towards enhanced metabolic flexibility, it's essential to cultivate a forward-looking perspective that embraces both progress and ongoing refinement.

1. **Continuous Self-Assessment:** Regularly assess your progress, not just in terms of physical changes but also in how you feel, your energy levels, and overall well-being. Use this self-reflection to make informed

adjustments to your diet, lifestyle, and exercise routine.

2. **Adaptability:** Recognize that your body's needs may evolve over time. Stay adaptable and be open to adjusting your dietary and lifestyle strategies accordingly. What works for you today may need modification as your goals, activity levels, and health status change.

3. **Goal Setting:** Establish clear and realistic goals for your metabolic flexibility journey. Whether your focus is on weight management, improved energy levels, or specific health markers, having defined goals provides direction and motivation.

4. **Celebrate Milestones:** Acknowledge and celebrate your achievements along the way. Whether it's reaching a fitness

milestone, maintaining a consistent dietary pattern, or overcoming a challenge, celebrating small victories reinforces positive habits.

5. **Educate Yourself:** Stay informed about advancements in nutrition, exercise science, and metabolic health. Knowledge empowers you to make informed choices and adapt your approach based on evolving insights in the field.

6. **Community Support:** Connect with others who share similar goals. Joining a community or finding a support network can provide motivation, shared experiences, and valuable insights. Social support can be a powerful catalyst for sustained progress.

7. **Professional Guidance:** Consider seeking guidance from healthcare

professionals, nutritionists, or fitness experts. Their expertise can offer personalized insights, address specific challenges, and optimize your approach based on individual factors.

8. **Mind-Body Connection:** Cultivate mindfulness in your approach to nutrition and physical activity. Pay attention to how different foods make you feel, listen to your body's hunger and fullness cues, and incorporate practices like meditation or yoga to enhance the mind-body connection.

9. **Experiment with Periodization:** Explore different phases of nutrition and exercise based on your goals. Periodizing your approach, such as alternating between higher and lower carbohydrate days, can provide

metabolic stimuli and prevent
adaptation.

10. **Long-Term Sustainability:**
    Strive for a metabolic flexibility
    lifestyle that is sustainable for the
    long term. Avoid extreme or
    restrictive approaches that may
    lead to burnout. Aim for a balance
    that aligns with your preferences,
    values, and overall well-being.

11. **Stay Curious:** Maintain a curious
    and exploratory mindset on your
    journey. Continuously learn about
    your body's responses to different
    stimuli, be it certain foods, types
    of exercise, or lifestyle practices.
    This curiosity fuels ongoing self-
    discovery.

12. **Celebrate Non-Physical
    Benefits:** While physical changes
    are often a goal, acknowledge and
    appreciate the non-physical
    benefits of your journey, such as

improved mood, enhanced mental clarity, or better sleep. These holistic improvements contribute to overall well-being.

As you look ahead on your metabolic flexibility journey, view it as an evolving adventure with opportunities for growth, learning, and self-improvement. Embrace the process, stay committed to your well-being, and enjoy the rewards of a resilient and adaptable metabolism.